BARIATRIC SURGERY MEAL PLAN

Comprehensive Guide Unlocking The Secrets To Post-Bariatric Surgery Success, Nourishing Meal Plans, Recipes And Practical Tips For Optimal Health And Wellness)

DR. ALLAN FREDA

Contents

Within the pages of this book, you'll discover a treasure trove of information curated to support your post-bariatric surgery journey.

From understanding the importance of nutrient-rich meals to crafting delicious and satisfying recipes, every aspect is meticulously crafted to empower you in your quest for wellness.

Proven tips are peppered throughout the book, offering invaluable insights garnered from experts and individuals who have walked this path before you. These tips serve as beacons of guidance, illuminating the way toward sustainable success.

So, whether you're just beginning your post-surgery chapter or seeking to enhance your current routine, this book is your trusted companion. It's more than just a collection of recipes; it's a holistic approach to nourishment, wellness, and ultimately, a fulfilling life beyond bariatric surgery.

Disclaimer

The information in this book is for informational purposes only and should not replace professional medical advice, diagnosis, or treatment. Always consult your physician or a qualified health provider regarding any medical concerns. Do not disregard professional medical advice or delay seeking it based on information in this book.

The author does not endorse or have affiliations with any mentioned entities. References are for informational purposes only.

Consult your healthcare provider before making dietary or lifestyle changes, especially during recovery from surgery, as individual needs vary.

Results may vary, and the information provided is not guaranteed to produce specific outcomes.

By reading this book, you acknowledge and agree to consult your healthcare provider before implementing any information herein.

For further guidance, consult your healthcare provider or reputable medical websites for reliable information on surgery recovery diets.

CHAPTER 1
UNDERSTANDING BARIATRIC SURGERY AND MEAL PLANNING

Bariatric surgery stands as a critical intervention for individuals grappling with severe obesity, offering a pathway to sustainable weight loss and improved health outcomes.

This surgical procedure, often considered a last resort after traditional weight loss methods have proven ineffective, involves altering the digestive system to restrict food intake and promote feelings of fullness.

It's crucial to comprehend the various aspects of bariatric surgery and its implications for meal planning to ensure the success of the procedure and long-term health benefits.

Bariatric surgery represents a significant step towards achieving weight loss and managing obesity-related health conditions.

This surgical approach aims to modify the gastrointestinal tract, typically by reducing the size of the stomach or rerouting the digestive system, thereby limiting the amount of food a person can consume and absorb. The ultimate goal of bariatric surgery is to induce weight loss, alleviate obesity-related health issues such as type 2 diabetes and hypertension, and enhance overall quality of life. While bariatric surgery is a highly effective intervention, it requires careful consideration and commitment from patients, including adherence to dietary guidelines post-surgery.

Types of Bariatric Surgery Procedures:

Several types of bariatric surgery procedures exist, each with its unique mechanisms and outcomes. The most common procedures include gastric bypass, sleeve gastrectomy, adjustable gastric banding, and biliopancreatic diversion with a duodenal switch. With a gastric bypass, the stomach's upper pouch is made smaller and the digestive juices are redirected.

small intestine to connect to this pouch, effectively bypassing a portion of the stomach and intestine. Sleeve gastrectomy entails removing a large portion of the stomach, leaving behind a narrow sleeve-like structure. Adjustable gastric banding involves placing a band around the upper part of the stomach to create a small pouch and restrict food intake.

Biliopancreatic diversion with duodenal switch combines restrictive and malabsorptive components by removing a portion of restricting food consumption and nutrient absorption by rerouting the small intestine and the stomach.

The choice of procedure depends on factors such as the patient's medical history, body mass index (BMI), and individual preferences.

Meal planning assumes paramount importance in the post-bariatric surgery phase to support recovery, promote weight loss, and prevent complications. Following bariatric surgery, the stomach's reduced size and altered digestive anatomy necessitate dietary modifications to accommodate these changes and ensure optimal nutrient intake.

A well-designed meal plan tailored to individual needs helps bariatric patients adjust to their new eating habits, control portion sizes, and make nutritious food choices. Moreover, proper meal planning can minimize the risk of complications such as dumping syndrome, nutrient deficiencies, and weight regain, which are common concerns following bariatric surgery. By adhering to a structured meal plan, patients can optimize their nutritional status, enhance satiety, and facilitate long-term weight management success.

Bariatric patients have unique nutritional requirements that must be addressed through a carefully crafted meal plan. Following surgery, individuals may experience reduced tolerance to certain foods, decreased appetite, and changes in nutrient absorption, necessitating a nutrient-dense diet that prioritizes protein, vitamins, and minerals.

Protein plays a crucial role in promoting wound healing, preserving lean muscle mass, and supporting metabolic function, making it an essential component of post-bariatric meal plans. Adequate hydration is also imperative to prevent dehydration and facilitate digestion, particularly considering the reduced stomach capacity post-surgery.

Additionally, bariatric patients must focus on consuming micronutrient-rich foods such as fruits, vegetables, and whole grains to meet their vitamin and mineral needs while minimizing the risk of deficiencies.

Regular monitoring of nutritional status and ongoing dietary counseling are integral aspects of post-bariatric care to ensure patients achieve and maintain optimal health outcomes.

Comprehensive Guide Unlocking the Secrets to Post-Bariatric Surgery Success, Nourishing Meal Plans, Recipes, and Practical Tips for Optimal Health and Wellness:

Embarking on the journey toward post-bariatric surgery success requires a comprehensive approach that encompasses meal planning, nutritional guidance, and lifestyle modifications. This guide serves as a roadmap for individuals navigating the challenges and opportunities associated with bariatric surgery, offering invaluable insights into crafting nourishing meal plans, preparing delicious recipes, and implementing practical tips for optimal health and wellness.

Achieving sustainable weight loss and maintaining long-term health following bariatric surgery necessitates unlocking the secrets to post-operative success. Beyond the surgical procedure itself, success hinges on adopting healthy eating habits, adhering to dietary guidelines, and making lifestyle changes conducive to weight management.

This entails understanding the physiological changes that occur post-surgery, including alterations in appetite, digestion, and nutrient absorption, and adjusting one's approach to food accordingly. By embracing a holistic approach to post-bariatric care, individuals can overcome challenges, harness the benefits of surgery, and embark on a journey toward improved health and well-being.

Central to post-bariatric surgery success is the development of nourishing meal plans that cater to individual nutritional needs, preferences, and goals. A well-balanced meal plan should prioritize lean protein sources, fibrous vegetables, whole grains, and healthy fats while limiting refined carbohydrates, sugars, and processed foods.

Portion control is paramount, given the reduced stomach capacity post-surgery, necessitating smaller, more frequent meals to prevent discomfort and promote satiety. Incorporating a variety of nutrient-dense foods ensures adequate intake of essential vitamins and minerals while supporting overall health and wellness. Meal planning strategies may include prepping meals in advance, portioning out servings, and incorporating diverse flavors and textures to enhance satisfaction and enjoyment.

Delicious and nutritious recipes form the cornerstone of a successful post-bariatric meal plan, offering a variety of options to suit individual tastes and dietary requirements. From protein-packed salads and stir-fries to hearty soups and casseroles, the possibilities are endless when it comes to creating satisfying meals that support weight loss and promote optimal health. Embracing whole, minimally processed ingredients allows individuals to maximize flavor and nutrition while minimizing empty calories and additives.

Experimenting with herbs, spices, and seasonings adds depth and complexity to dishes without compromising their nutritional integrity. Whether seeking quick and easy weeknight dinners or indulgent yet guilt-free treats, a collection of carefully curated recipes empowers individuals to stay on track with their post-bariatric meal plan while enjoying delicious and satisfying meals.

In addition to meal planning and recipe selection, incorporating practical tips for optimal health and wellness enhances the post-bariatric surgery experience and promotes long-term success. Strategies may include mindful eating practices such as chewing slowly, Savoring each bite, and listening to hunger and fullness cues to prevent overeating. Regular physical activity is also crucial for supporting weight loss, improving metabolic health, and enhancing overall well-being. Whether engaging in structured exercise routines, incorporating daily movement into one's lifestyle, or exploring enjoyable recreational activities, finding ways to stay active promotes adherence to healthy habits and facilitates weight maintenance. Furthermore, prioritizing self-care practices such as adequate sleep, stress management, and social support fosters emotional resilience and enhances the overall quality of life post-bariatric surgery.

By embracing a holistic approach to health and wellness, individuals can unlock their full potential and thrive in their post-operative journey toward a healthier, happier life.

CHAPTER 2
GETTING STARTED WITH MEAL PREP

Meal planning and preparation are crucial aspects of post-bariatric surgery success, facilitating optimal health and wellness. This comprehensive guide will unlock the secrets to effective meal planning, providing nourishing meal plans, recipes, and practical tips to support your journey towards optimal health and wellness.

Essential Kitchen Tools and Equipment

Equipping your kitchen with essential tools and equipment lays the foundation for successful meal preparation post-bariatric surgery. Invest in quality kitchen tools such as sharp knives, cutting boards, measuring cups and spoons, mixing bowls, pots, and pans. These tools not only streamline the cooking process but also ensure precision in portion control, a key aspect of post-bariatric meal planning. Additionally, consider investing in kitchen appliances such as a blender, food processor, and slow cooker, which can simplify the preparation of nutritious meals while preserving essential nutrients. Having these tools readily available empowers you to create delicious and healthy meals tailored to your post-bariatric dietary needs.

Stocking Your Pantry and Fridge

Stocking your pantry and fridge with nutritious staples is essential for maintaining a post-bariatric surgery meal plan. Focus on incorporating lean proteins such as chicken, turkey, fish, tofu, and legumes, which are vital for muscle repair and metabolism. Opt for whole grains like quinoa, brown rice, and oats, which provide sustained energy and fiber to support digestive health.

Include a variety of fruits and vegetables, both fresh and frozen, to ensure a diverse nutrient intake.

Be mindful of added sugars and processed foods, opting instead for whole food options to support your weight loss and health goals.

Additionally, ensure your pantry is stocked with herbs, spices, and condiments to enhance the flavor of your meals without relying on excess salt or sugar.

Meal Planning Basics

Effective meal planning is the cornerstone of post-bariatric surgery success, enabling you to meet your nutritional needs while adhering to dietary guidelines. Begin by setting aside dedicated time each week to plan your meals and snacks, taking into account your nutritional requirements and personal preferences. Start by outlining your meals for the week, considering a balance of lean proteins, complex carbohydrates, and healthy fats.

Incorporate a variety of flavors and textures to keep meals interesting and satisfying. Utilize online resources, cookbooks, and meal-planning apps to find inspiration and streamline the planning process.

Additionally, consider batch-cooking large quantities of staples such as grains, proteins, and vegetables to simplify meal assembly throughout the week.

Flexibility is key to successful meal planning, so don't hesitate to adjust your plan based on changing circumstances or preferences.

Tips for Successful Meal Prepping

Efficient meal prepping is essential for maintaining consistency and adherence to your post-bariatric surgery meal plan. Start by designating a specific day each week for meal prep, allowing ample time to cook and portion out your meals and snacks. Invest in quality storage containers to keep prepared meals fresh and organized throughout the week. Prioritize perishable items and ingredients that require longer cooking times to ensure optimal freshness and flavor. Consider preparing versatile components such as grilled chicken breast, roasted vegetables, and cooked grains, which can be easily incorporated into various meals. Embrace variety by experimenting with different recipes, flavors, and cuisines to prevent boredom and monotony. Remember to include healthy snacks and portable options for busy days or on-the-go convenience. Lastly, practice mindful portion control to avoid overeating and support your weight loss goals.

By equipping your kitchen with essential tools, stocking your pantry with nutritious staples, mastering the basics of meal planning, and implementing effective meal-prepping strategies, you can unlock the secrets to post-bariatric surgery success. Nourishing meal plans, recipes, and practical tips will empower you to prioritize your health and wellness, ensuring optimal outcomes on your journey toward a healthier lifestyle.

CHAPTER 3
BREAKFAST DELIGHTS

Breakfast is often touted as the most important meal of the day, and for individuals who have undergone bariatric surgery, it becomes even more crucial. A well-balanced breakfast sets the tone for the day, providing essential nutrients and energy to kickstart metabolism and support weight loss efforts.

However, post-bariatric surgery patients face unique dietary challenges, requiring careful consideration of portion sizes, nutrient density, and meal composition. In this comprehensive guide, we delve into the intricacies of crafting a bariatric surgery meal plan tailored specifically for breakfast, offering a variety of protein-packed delights, low-carb options, energizing smoothie recipes, and convenient make-ahead breakfast casseroles to unlock the secrets to post-bariatric surgery success and foster optimal health and wellness.

Protein is the cornerstone of a bariatric surgery meal plan, playing a pivotal role in muscle repair, satiety, and metabolic function. Following surgery, patients often have increased protein requirements to support healing and weight loss.

Therefore, incorporating protein-rich foods into breakfast is essential for meeting these needs and promoting long-term success. Opt for lean sources of protein such as eggs, Greek yogurt, cottage cheese, turkey bacon, and tofu.

Consider preparing scrambled eggs with vegetables, Greek yogurt parfaits with berries and nuts, turkey bacon avocado wraps, or tofu scramble with spinach and mushrooms. These protein-packed breakfast ideas not only provide essential amino acids but also help control hunger and stabilize blood sugar levels throughout the morning.

Reducing carbohydrate intake is a common strategy employed post-bariatric surgery to facilitate weight loss and prevent dumping syndrome.

While carbohydrates are not inherently bad, selecting complex carbohydrates with high fiber content and low glycemic index is advisable. When planning breakfast, focus on incorporating nutrient-dense, low-carb options such as leafy greens, cruciferous vegetables, berries, nuts, seeds, and whole grains in moderation.

Swap traditional carb-heavy breakfast staples like pancakes, waffles, and sugary cereals for healthier alternatives such as vegetable omelettes, chia seed pudding, avocado toast on whole grain bread, or almond flour pancakes topped with Greek yogurt and berries.

These low-carb breakfast options provide sustained energy without the risk of blood sugar spikes or excessive calorie intake.

Smoothies are a convenient and versatile breakfast option for bariatric surgery patients, especially in the early stages of recovery when solid foods may be challenging to tolerate. Blending nutrient-rich ingredients into a delicious and satisfying beverage allows for easy digestion and absorption of essential nutrients. When creating energizing smoothie recipes, aim to include a balance of protein, healthy fats, fiber, and carbohydrates to promote satiety and stabilize blood sugar levels.

Combine ingredients such as protein powder, leafy greens, unsweetened almond milk, avocado, berries, and flaxseed or chia seeds. Experiment with different flavor combinations like chocolate banana, green goddess, tropical paradise, or berry blast to keep breakfast exciting and enjoyable. These energizing smoothie recipes offer a refreshing way to start the day while nourishing the body with essential vitamins, minerals, and antioxidants.

Make-Ahead Breakfast Casseroles:
For busy mornings or hectic schedules, make-ahead breakfast casseroles are a lifesaver for bariatric surgery patients seeking convenience without sacrificing nutritional quality. These hearty and satisfying dishes can be prepared in advance and portioned out for quick and easy meals throughout the week.

When assembling breakfast casseroles, focus on incorporating a balance of protein, vegetables, and healthy fats to create a well-rounded dish.

Use ingredients such as eggs, lean meats, spinach, bell peppers, onions, cheese, and whole-grain bread or tortillas. Prepare variations such as crustless quiches, egg muffins, or breakfast burrito casseroles that can be customized to suit individual preferences and dietary restrictions.

By batch cooking these make-ahead breakfast casseroles, patients can streamline their morning routine and ensure they have nutritious options readily available to support their post-bariatric surgery journey toward optimal health and wellness.

CHAPTER 4
LUNCHTIME FAVORITES

Lunchtime is a crucial part of the day for anyone, especially for those who have undergone bariatric surgery. It's essential to refuel the body with nutrient-rich meals that support healing, weight loss, and overall health. In this section, we'll explore various lunchtime favorites tailored specifically for individuals who have had bariatric surgery.

From protein-rich salad recipes to satisfying soup and stew options, creative sandwich and wrap ideas to quick and easy lunchbox meals, we'll unlock the secrets to post-bariatric surgery success through nourishing meal plans, recipes, and practical tips for optimal health and wellness.

Protein-Rich Salad Recipes

Salads are a fantastic lunch option for bariatric surgery patients as they are typically light, yet packed with essential nutrients, especially protein. Protein is crucial post-surgery as it aids in healing and helps maintain muscle mass while promoting satiety, ultimately supporting weight loss.

When crafting protein-rich salad recipes, opt for lean protein sources such as grilled chicken, turkey, tofu, or beans. Incorporate a variety of colorful vegetables for added vitamins, minerals, and fiber, which promote digestion and overall gut health. Consider adding a source of healthy fat like avocado or nuts to enhance flavor and increase satiety.

Dress salads with homemade vinaigrettes or low-fat dressings to control added sugars and unnecessary calories. Experiment with different combinations of ingredients to keep salads exciting and enjoyable, ensuring that patients stay on track with their post-bariatric surgery meal plan.

Soups and stews are not only comforting and delicious but also convenient and easy to prepare, making them ideal for bariatric surgery patients during lunchtime.

These dishes can be packed with protein, vegetables, and complex carbohydrates, providing a well-rounded meal that supports post-surgery nutritional needs. Opt for broth-based soups or stews rather than cream-based ones to reduce excess calories and fat while still delivering robust flavor. Incorporate lean protein sources such as chicken, turkey, fish, or legumes to promote satiety and muscle recovery. Load up on vegetables like carrots, celery, spinach, and kale to boost fiber intake and enhance nutrient density.

Experiment with herbs, spices, and low-sodium broths to add depth and complexity to soups and stews without compromising on flavor. Prepare large batches ahead of time and portion them out for easy grab-and-go lunches throughout the week, ensuring that bariatric surgery patients have nutritious options readily available to support their journey toward optimal health and wellness.

Sandwiches and wraps are classic lunchtime staples that can easily be adapted to fit into a bariatric surgery meal plan. By choosing the right ingredients and portion sizes, patients can enjoy satisfying and flavorful sandwiches and wraps that align with their dietary needs and goals.

Opt for whole-grain bread or wraps to increase fiber intake and promote satiety while providing essential nutrients like vitamins, minerals, and antioxidants. Choose lean protein options such as grilled chicken, turkey, or tuna salad made with Greek yogurt instead of mayonnaise to keep fat and calorie content in check. Load up sandwiches and wraps with plenty of vegetables like lettuce, tomatoes, cucumbers, and bell peppers to add volume, texture, and flavor without excess calories. Experiment with different spreads and condiments like hummus, pesto, or mustard to enhance taste while keeping added sugars and unhealthy fats to a minimum. Get creative with flavor combinations and ingredients to keep sandwiches and wraps exciting and enjoyable, ensuring that bariatric surgery patients stay satisfied and on track with their post-surgery meal plan.

For bariatric surgery patients on the go, quick and easy lunchbox meals are a convenient and practical option to ensure they stay nourished and energized throughout the day. By preparing meals ahead of time and portioning them out into grab-and-go containers, patients can save time and effort while still enjoying nutritious and satisfying lunches. Focus on incorporating a balance of protein, vegetables, healthy fats, and complex carbohydrates to provide sustained energy and promote satiety. Consider meal-prepping staples like grilled chicken, quinoa, roasted vegetables, and mixed greens to have on hand for assembling quick and easy lunchbox meals.

Pack snacks like Greek yogurt, nuts, seeds, or fresh fruit to round out meals and provide additional nutrients and variety. Invest in insulated lunch bags or bento boxes to keep meals fresh and safe to eat, especially if patients don't have access to refrigeration throughout the day. By prioritizing preparation and planning, bariatric surgery patients can maintain a consistent and nutritious eating routine, supporting their long-term success and well-being post-surgery.

CHAPTER 5
DELICIOUS DINNERS

In the journey towards post-bariatric surgery success, establishing a well-structured meal plan is essential for achieving optimal health and wellness. One of the pivotal components of such a plan is crafting delicious and nourishing dinners that cater to the specific dietary needs of individuals who have undergone bariatric surgery. These dinners not only need to be flavorful and satisfying but also balanced in nutrients to support the body's healing and weight management process.

Flavorful Protein Entrees: Protein plays a crucial role in the post-bariatric surgery meal plan as it aids in muscle repair, supports satiety, and helps maintain metabolic function. Flavorful protein entrees serve as the centrepiece of dinner meals, providing the necessary building blocks for the body's tissues and cells.

Opting for lean protein sources such as grilled chicken, turkey, fish, tofu, or legumes ensures a low-fat intake while maximizing protein content. Incorporating various cooking methods like grilling, baking, or sautéing allows for versatility in flavors and textures, keeping the dinner options exciting and satisfying.

Veggie-Packed Side Dishes: Incorporating ample servings of vegetables into dinner meals is essential for providing essential vitamins, minerals, and fiber while keeping calorie intake in check.

Veggie-packed side dishes complement protein entrees, adding color, texture, and nutritional value to the meal. Steamed, roasted, or stir-fried vegetables such as broccoli, cauliflower, spinach, bell peppers, and zucchini offer a spectrum of flavors and nutrients without adding excess calories or fat. Experimenting with herbs, spices, and healthy cooking oils enhances the taste and appeal of vegetable side dishes, making them a delicious and satisfying component of the bariatric surgery meal plan.

One-Pan Dinner Recipes: Streamlining the dinner preparation process is particularly beneficial for individuals following a post-bariatric surgery meal plan, where convenience and efficiency are paramount.

One-pan dinner recipes simplify cooking and cleanup while offering a balanced combination of protein, vegetables, and grains in a single dish. Meals like sheet pan chicken with roasted vegetables, shrimp stir-fry with quinoa, or baked fish with Mediterranean vegetables minimize the need for extensive meal planning and preparation, making it easier to adhere to dietary guidelines without sacrificing flavor or nutrition.

Comforting Casseroles and Bakes: Comfort foods hold a special place in many people's hearts, providing a sense of familiarity and satisfaction during mealtime.

However, traditional casseroles and bakes often contain high amounts of refined carbohydrates and fats, which may not align with the dietary goals of individuals post-bariatric surgery.

By reinventing classic recipes with nutrient-dense ingredients and mindful portion control, comforting casseroles and bakes can be transformed into nourishing dinner options that support post-surgery health and wellness.

Utilizing whole grains, lean proteins, and plenty of vegetables, recipes like turkey and vegetable quinoa bake, spaghetti squash lasagna, or Mexican cauliflower rice casserole offer the warmth and flavor of traditional comfort foods without compromising on nutritional integrity.

crafting delicious and nourishing dinners is a cornerstone of post-bariatric surgery meal planning, contributing to long-term success and well-being.

By focusing on flavorful protein entrees, veggie-packed side dishes, one-pan dinner recipes, and comforting casseroles and bakes, individuals can unlock the secrets to post-surgery success while enjoying a variety of satisfying meals that promote optimal health and wellness.

CHAPTER 6
SNACKS AND APPETIZERS

After undergoing bariatric surgery, it's crucial to adhere to a well-balanced meal plan to support your body's healing process and promote sustainable weight loss. Snacks and appetizers play a significant role in maintaining energy levels throughout the day and preventing overeating during main meals. By focusing on nutrient-dense options and portion control, you can ensure that your snacks contribute to your overall health and wellness goals.

Portable Protein Snacks

Protein is essential for muscle repair, satiety, and overall metabolic function, making it a cornerstone of post-bariatric surgery nutrition. Portable protein snacks offer convenience and versatility, allowing you to meet your protein needs even when you're on the go. Opt for options such as beef jerky, hard-boiled eggs, Greek yogurt cups, string cheese, or protein bars specifically formulated for bariatric patients. These snacks are not only convenient but also help you stay on track with your protein intake goals, supporting your body's healing and weight loss journey.

Appetizers are often associated with indulgence, but post-bariatric surgery, it's essential to prioritize nutrient density and portion control. Guilt-free appetizers can satisfy cravings while still aligning with your dietary requirements. Consider options like vegetable crudites with hummus, shrimp cocktail, smoked salmon roll-ups, or caprese skewers with cherry tomatoes, mozzarella, and basil. These appetizers are low in calories and high in nutrients, allowing you to enjoy them without derailing your progress or compromising your health goals.

Dips can add flavor and texture to snacks and appetizers, but they often come with hidden calories and unhealthy fats.

However, with the right ingredients and preparation methods, you can create nutrient-dense dip recipes that enhance the nutritional value of your meals. Experiment with homemade guacamole made from ripe avocados, salsa fresca with fresh tomatoes and cilantro, Greek yogurt tzatziki with cucumber and dill, or black bean dip seasoned with lime and cumin. These dips are rich in vitamins, minerals, and fiber, providing a satisfying and nourishing addition to your snack repertoire.

Crunchy and crispy snacks are satisfying to eat and can help curb cravings for less healthy options like chips and crackers. However, post-bariatric surgery, it's important to choose snacks that are both satisfying and nutritious.

Consider alternatives such as roasted chickpeas seasoned with spices, kale chips tossed in olive oil and sea salt, air-popped popcorn sprinkled with nutritional yeast, or baked sweet potato fries served with a side of Greek yogurt dip. These snacks provide a satisfying crunch while delivering essential nutrients, fiber, and antioxidants to support your overall health and wellness.

Incorporating a variety of snacks and appetizers into your post-bariatric surgery meal plan can help you stay satisfied, energized, and on track with your health and wellness goals. By focusing on portable protein snacks, guilt-free appetizers, nutrient-dense dip recipes, and crunchy and crispy snack ideas, you can create a balanced and nourishing eating plan that supports your body's healing and promotes long-term success. Experiment with different ingredients and flavors to keep your meals exciting and enjoyable while prioritizing your health and well-being.

CHAPTER 7
SWEET TREATS AND DESSERTS

Sweet treats and desserts hold a unique place in our culinary culture, often associated with indulgence and celebration. However, for individuals who have undergone bariatric surgery, navigating the world of desserts can be challenging due to the need to maintain a balanced and nutritious diet while managing portion sizes and avoiding excessive sugars and fats. In this comprehensive guide to post-bariatric surgery success, we'll delve into the concept of creating bariatric-friendly sweet treats and desserts, offering nourishing meal plans, recipes, and practical tips for optimal health and wellness.

Decadent Desserts with a Healthy Twist: Decadent desserts need not be off-limits for individuals who have undergone bariatric surgery.

By incorporating healthier ingredients and mindful portion control, it is possible to enjoy sweet treats without compromising one's dietary goals.

One approach to creating decadent desserts with a healthy twist is to focus on natural sweeteners such as stevia, erythritol, or monk fruit extract instead of refined sugars. These alternatives provide sweetness without causing spikes in blood sugar levels, making them suitable for those with diabetes or insulin resistance, common concerns among bariatric surgery patients.

Additionally, utilizing whole food ingredients such as fruits, nuts, and seeds can add both flavor and nutritional value to desserts, boosting their fiber and nutrient content. For example, a decadent chocolate avocado mousse can satisfy cravings for rich, creamy desserts while providing heart-healthy fats and antioxidants. By experimenting with different flavor combinations and ingredient substitutions, individuals can indulge in their favorite desserts while supporting their post-bariatric surgery dietary needs.

Sugar-Free and Low-Carb Dessert Recipes: Sugar-free and low-carb dessert recipes are particularly well-suited for individuals following a bariatric surgery meal plan, as they help regulate blood sugar levels and promote weight loss or maintenance. These recipes often utilize alternative sweeteners such as stevia, erythritol, or xylitol, which have minimal impact on blood glucose levels and caloric intake. Common ingredients in sugar-free and low-carb desserts include almond flour, coconut flour, and flaxseed meal, which provide texture and structure without the need for traditional wheat flour. Additionally, incorporating high-protein ingredients such as Greek yogurt, cottage cheese, or protein powder can increase satiety and support muscle repair and growth, essential considerations for bariatric surgery patients. Examples of sugar-free and low-carb desserts include berry chia seed pudding, almond flour brownies, and coconut flour pancakes, all of which offer sweetness and satisfaction without the drawbacks of refined sugars and excessive carbohydrates. By embracing these recipes, individuals can enjoy delicious desserts while adhering to their post-bariatric surgery dietary guidelines.

Indulgent Treats in Moderation: While moderation is key to maintaining a healthy diet after bariatric surgery, indulgent treats can still have a place in one's meal plan when consumed mindfully and in appropriate portions.

Rather than eliminating treats such as chocolate, cookies, or ice cream, individuals can incorporate them into their diet in controlled amounts, allowing for enjoyment without derailing progress. Portion control is crucial when indulging in treats, as even small servings can contribute significant calories and sugar. For example, opting for a single serving of dark chocolate or a small scoop of high-protein ice cream can satisfy cravings without exceeding calorie or carbohydrate limits. Additionally, pairing indulgent treats with nutrient-dense foods such as fruits, nuts, or yogurt can help balance blood sugar levels and increase satiety, reducing the risk of overeating.

By approaching indulgent treats with mindfulness and moderation, individuals can maintain a healthy relationship with food while supporting their post-bariatric surgery goals.

Homemade Protein Bars and Bites: Homemade protein bars and bites are convenient, portable snacks that can provide a quick and satisfying energy boost while supporting post-bariatric surgery dietary requirements. Unlike commercial protein bars, which may contain artificial additives, excessive sugars, or preservatives, homemade versions allow for full control over ingredients and nutritional content. When crafting homemade protein bars and bites, it's essential to prioritize high-quality protein sources such as whey protein powder, collagen peptides, or plant-based protein sources like hemp or pea protein. Protein is essential for supporting muscle repair and metabolism, making it a crucial component of the post-bariatric surgery diet. Additionally, incorporating healthy fats from sources like nuts, seeds, or nut butter can enhance flavor and satiety while providing essential nutrients such as omega-3 fatty acids and vitamin E. By experimenting with different flavor combinations and textures, individuals can create customized protein bars and bites that align with their taste preferences and nutritional needs. Whether enjoyed as a snack between meals or as a post-workout refuel, homemade protein bars and bites offer a convenient and nutritious option for bariatric surgery patients striving for optimal health and wellness.

CHAPTER 8
SPECIAL OCCASION FEASTS

In the journey of post-bariatric surgery, special occasions such as festive holidays, elegant dinner parties, and celebratory gatherings pose unique challenges. However, with thoughtful planning and consideration, these occasions can still be enjoyed while adhering to your bariatric meal plan. Here, we delve into the strategies and ideas for navigating special occasion feasts post-bariatric surgery, ensuring you can partake in the joy of these events without compromising your health goals.

Festive Holiday Menus

During festive holidays, food often takes center stage, presenting an array of tempting dishes that may not align with your bariatric meal plan. However, with strategic menu planning, you can create festive holiday menus that are both delicious and bariatric-friendly.

Opt for protein-rich main courses such as roasted turkey or baked salmon, accompanied by nutrient-dense sides like roasted vegetables or quinoa salad. Incorporating colorful fruits and vegetables not only adds flavor and variety but also boosts nutritional value. Additionally, consider healthier cooking methods such as grilling, baking, or steaming to minimize added fats and calories.

By focusing on wholesome ingredients and mindful portion control, you can savor the holiday season without derailing your progress.

Elegant Dinner Party Ideas

Hosting or attending an elegant dinner party post-bariatric surgery requires careful planning to ensure both sophistication and adherence to your dietary restrictions. When crafting your menu, prioritize protein-rich dishes such as grilled chicken skewers, shrimp cocktails, or lean beef tenderloin.

Pair these protein options with flavorful vegetable sides or salads, incorporating a variety of textures and colors to elevate the dining experience.

For dessert, consider lighter options such as fruit sorbet, yogurt parfaits, or dark chocolate-dipped strawberries to satisfy your sweet cravings without excessive sugar or calories. Furthermore, focus on creating an inviting atmosphere with elegant table settings and thoughtful décor to enhance the overall dining experience for you and your guests.

Indulging in celebratory cakes and desserts post-bariatric surgery can be challenging, given their typically high sugar and calorie content. However, with the right recipes and modifications, you can enjoy delicious treats without compromising your dietary goals. Opt for lighter dessert options such as flourless chocolate cake, protein-packed cheesecake bites, or fruit-based desserts like grilled peaches with cinnamon yogurt sauce.

 Experiment with alternative sweeteners such as stevia or monk fruit to reduce sugar content while still satisfying your sweet tooth. Additionally, focus on portion control and mindful eating to prevent overindulgence, Savoring each bite and appreciating the flavors without guilt.

Tips for Dining Out Post-Surgery

Dining out post-bariatric surgery requires careful consideration to navigate restaurant menus and make healthy choices. Begin by researching restaurants in advance and reviewing their menus online to identify bariatric-friendly options.

Look for dishes that are grilled, baked, or steamed rather than fried or sautéed, and request modifications such as substituting vegetables for starches or sauces on the side. Additionally, prioritize protein-rich entrees such as grilled fish, chicken breast, or lean cuts of meat, and complement them with nutrient-dense sides such as steamed vegetables or salad. Practice portion control by opting for appetizer-sized portions or sharing entrees with dining companions to avoid overeating. Finally, listen to your body's hunger and fullness cues, stopping eating when satisfied rather than finishing everything on your plate. With mindful choices and preparation, dining out can be an enjoyable and satisfying experience while supporting your post-bariatric surgery journey.

CHAPTER 9
BEVERAGE SELECTIONS

Bariatric surgery is a life-changing procedure that requires careful attention to post-operative dietary habits, including beverage choices. Hydration becomes particularly important after bariatric surgery, as the body's ability to absorb nutrients may be altered. Therefore, selecting appropriate beverages is crucial for maintaining optimal health and supporting weight loss goals. In this section, we will explore hydration tips tailored for bariatric patients, provide low-calorie drink recipes to support their nutritional needs, and offer ideas for mocktails

and cocktails (in moderation) to add variety to their beverage options while still adhering to their dietary guidelines.

Proper hydration is essential for overall health, but it becomes even more critical for individuals who have undergone bariatric surgery. After surgery, the stomach's capacity is significantly reduced, which means that patients may not be able to consume large quantities of fluids at once. As a result, bariatric patients need to sip fluids throughout the day to stay adequately hydrated.

Opting for hydrating beverages that provide essential electrolytes without adding excess calories or sugar is key. Water should be the primary beverage choice, as it hydrates the body without adding extra calories or sugar. Infusing water with fruits, such as lemon or berries, can enhance its flavor without compromising its nutritional value. Additionally, sugar-free flavored water or herbal teas can provide variety without contributing to calorie intake. Bariatric patients must avoid sugary drinks, such as soda or fruit juice, as they can lead to dumping syndrome or hinder weight loss progress. Monitoring urine color can also serve as a helpful indicator of hydration status; pale yellow urine suggests adequate hydration, while darker urine may indicate dehydration. Overall, prioritizing hydration through consistent, low-calorie beverage consumption is essential for bariatric patients to support their health and recovery journey.

Low-Calorie Drink Recipes

Creating delicious and nutritious beverages that align with bariatric dietary guidelines can enhance the post-operative experience for patients. Incorporating nutrient-dense ingredients into drink recipes ensures that patients receive essential vitamins and minerals without excess calories or sugar. One option is a green smoothie made with spinach or kale, non-fat Greek yogurt, and a small amount of fruit for sweetness. This smoothie provides a boost of protein and fiber while keeping the calorie count low. Another option is a protein shake made with unsweetened almond milk, protein powder, and a tablespoon of nut butter for added flavor and satiety. For a refreshing alternative to plain water, patients can try infused water recipes using cucumber, mint, and lime for a burst of flavor without added calories. Additionally, homemade vegetable juices, such as carrot or beet juice, can provide essential nutrients while keeping calorie intake in check. Experimenting with different ingredients and flavors allows bariatric patients to enjoy a diverse range of low-calorie beverages that support their nutritional needs and promote weight loss success.

Mocktail and Cocktail Ideas (in Moderation)
While alcohol consumption should be limited after bariatric surgery due to its high-calorie content and potential for nutrient malabsorption, enjoying an occasional mocktail or cocktail in moderation can be a part of a balanced lifestyle for some patients. Mocktails, or non-alcoholic cocktails, offer the opportunity to enjoy flavorful beverages

without the added calories or risks associated with alcohol consumption.

For example, a virgin mojito made with club soda, fresh mint, lime juice, and a splash of agave syrup provides a refreshing alternative to traditional cocktails. Similarly, a mocktail mimicking a margarita can be made using fresh citrus juices, agave syrup, and a salt rim for added authenticity. When consuming alcoholic beverages, moderation is key.

Bariatric patients should be mindful of portion sizes and choose lower-calorie options, such as light beer or wine spritzers, to minimize calorie intake. It's also important to consume alcohol slowly and with food to reduce the risk of complications, such as dumping syndrome or alcohol intolerance.

By incorporating mocktails and cocktails into their diet in moderation, bariatric patients can enjoy social occasions while still adhering to their dietary guidelines and supporting their weight loss goals.

 selecting appropriate beverages is crucial for bariatric patients to support their health and weight loss journey post-surgery. Prioritizing hydration through consistent low-calorie beverage consumption, such as water infused with fruits or herbal teas, ensures that patients stay adequately hydrated without compromising their nutritional goals. Incorporating nutrient-dense ingredients into drink recipes allows patients to enjoy delicious and satisfying beverages that support their nutritional needs while promoting weight loss success. Additionally, enjoying mocktails and cocktails in moderation can add variety to the diet without derailing progress. By making mindful beverage choices, bariatric patients can optimize their health and well-being following surgery.

CHAPTER 10
MAINTAINING SUCCESS AND LONG-TERM WELLNESS

Bariatric surgery is a life-altering procedure that requires significant commitment and lifestyle changes to achieve long-term success and wellness. While the surgery itself can jumpstart weight loss, sustaining these results requires adherence to a well-structured bariatric surgery meal plan and the adoption of healthy habits. This comprehensive guide aims to unlock the secrets to post-bariatric surgery success, offering nourishing meal plans, recipes, and practical tips for optimal health and wellness.

Strategies for Long-Term Success:
Long-term success after bariatric surgery hinges on implementing effective strategies that support sustained weight loss and overall well-being.

One crucial aspect is adopting a balanced and nutritious meal plan tailored to meet the specific needs of post-bariatric surgery patients. Such a plan typically emphasizes high-protein, low-carbohydrate foods to promote satiety, preserve muscle mass, and prevent nutrient deficiencies. Additionally, portion control is paramount to prevent overeating and ensure weight maintenance. Regular monitoring of food intake, keeping a food diary, and attending support group meetings can help individuals stay accountable and motivated on their journey to long-term success.

Furthermore, cultivating a supportive environment and seeking professional guidance from dietitians or nutritionists can provide invaluable support in navigating dietary challenges and making sustainable lifestyle changes. These professionals can offer personalized recommendations, address nutritional deficiencies, and assist in meal planning to optimize outcomes post-surgery. Moreover, integrating mindfulness techniques into daily routines, such as mindful eating practices, can enhance self-awareness, improve eating behaviors, and promote healthier relationships with food.

While bariatric surgery can yield remarkable results, individuals may encounter challenges and plateaus along their weight loss journey. It's essential to anticipate and address these obstacles proactively to prevent setbacks and maintain momentum toward long-term success.

Common challenges post-surgery includes dealing with food cravings, emotional eating, and navigating social situations that revolve around food. Developing coping strategies, such as seeking alternative activities to cope with emotions or practicing stress-relief techniques like meditation, can help individuals manage triggers and prevent relapse into unhealthy eating habits.

Plateaus, where weight loss stalls despite adherence to dietary and exercise regimens, are also a common concern.

In such instances, reassessing dietary habits, increasing physical activity levels, and consulting with healthcare professionals can provide insights into potential barriers to progress. Adjustments to the meal plan, such as modifying macronutrient ratios or incorporating new foods, may be necessary to break through plateaus and reignite weight loss. Additionally, focusing on non-scale victories, such as improvements in energy levels, physical fitness, and overall well-being, can help individuals stay motivated during challenging times.

Regular physical activity is integral to long-term success after bariatric surgery, contributing to weight maintenance, muscle preservation, and overall health. However, initiating and maintaining an exercise routine post-surgery can be daunting for some individuals. It's essential to start gradually and choose activities that are enjoyable, sustainable, and aligned with individual fitness levels and preferences. Incorporating a combination of aerobic exercises, strength training, and flexibility exercises can provide comprehensive benefits, including improved cardiovascular health, increased metabolism, and enhanced mood.

Prioritizing consistency over intensity and setting realistic goals can help individuals establish a sustainable exercise routine. Try to get in at least 150 minutes of moderate-to-intense aerobic exercise or 75 minutes of intense exercise.

activity per week, as recommended by guidelines from organizations such as the American Heart Association. Additionally, incorporating strength training exercises two to three times per week can help preserve lean muscle mass and promote fat loss. Finding social support through group fitness classes, workout buddies, or online communities can also enhance motivation and accountability.

Mindful eating involves cultivating awareness and attention to the sensory experience of eating, including the taste, texture, and smell of food, as well as internal hunger and satiety cues.

This practice can help individuals develop a healthier relationship with food, improve eating behaviors, and prevent overeating. Post-bariatric surgery patients can benefit greatly from mindful eating practices, as they learn to reconnect with their bodies' signals of hunger and fullness, which may have been distorted by years of unhealthy eating habits.

To incorporate mindful eating into daily life, start by eating slowly, Savoring each bite, and paying attention to hunger and fullness cues. Minimize distractions during meals, such as television or electronic devices, to focus on the eating experience fully. Additionally, practicing portion control and stopping when satisfied, rather than overly full, can prevent discomfort and support weight management.

Mindfulness techniques, such as deep breathing or meditation, can also help individuals become more attuned to their bodies' signals and reduce emotional eating triggers.

maintaining success and long-term wellness after bariatric surgery requires a multifaceted approach that encompasses dietary adherence, regular physical activity, and mindful eating practices. By implementing strategies for long-term success, overcoming challenges and plateaus, incorporating exercise into daily routines, and practicing mindful eating, individuals can optimize their health and well-being post-surgery. With dedication, support, and guidance from healthcare professionals, achieving and sustaining optimal outcomes is within reach for those embarking on the transformative journey of bariatric surgery.

CONCLUSION

embarking on the journey of post-bariatric surgery success requires a comprehensive understanding of both the surgical process and the essential role of nutrition in achieving optimal health and wellness. Through diligent meal planning and preparation, individuals can unlock the secrets to long-term success and well-being.

Beginning with a solid foundation of knowledge about bariatric surgery procedures and the importance of post-surgery meal planning, individuals can then utilize practical tips and recipes provided in this guide to navigate their dietary journey effectively.

From protein-packed breakfasts to delicious dinners and indulgent desserts, each chapter offers a wealth of nourishing meal options designed to support the unique nutritional needs of bariatric patients.

With a focus on balance, variety, and portion control, these recipes empower individuals to enjoy flavorful meals while maintaining their weight loss goals. Moreover, this guide extends beyond the kitchen, addressing strategies for long-term success, overcoming challenges, and incorporating exercise and mindful eating practices into daily life.

By adopting a holistic approach to health and wellness, individuals can not only achieve their weight loss goals but also cultivate a sustainable lifestyle that promotes overall well-being.

In essence, this comprehensive guide serves as a roadmap for individuals embarking on their post-bariatric surgery journey, offering practical tools, nourishing meal plans, and invaluable insights to support their quest for optimal health and wellness. Through dedication, perseverance, and a commitment to self-care, individuals can unlock the full potential of their post-surgery experience and embrace a life of vitality and vitality.